EFFECTIVE WEIGHT LOSS BOOK FOR WOMEN OVER 40: A DIET AND EXERCISE GUIDE

George C. Hoffman

Table of contents

Introduction

A healthy and effective weight reduction diet for ladies ought to mean to make a calorie shortfall while as yet giving satisfactory nourishment and energy to help day to day exercises and exercise.

Keep in mind, weight reduction is a progressive cycle, and it's vital to be patient and steady with your eating regimen and exercise propensities.

Here are a few overall principles for a healthy and effective weight reduction diet and exercise:

Section 1

As we age, our digestion normally dials back, making it harder to lose weight. Nonetheless, ordinary activity can assist with helping digestion, increment muscle mass, and burn calories. Here are some effective weight reduction practices for ladies above 40:

Cardiovascular activities: These activities increment pulse and consume calories, like strolling, running, cycling, swimming, or moving. Aim for at least 150 minutes of moderate-force or 75 minutes of energetic power vigorous activity each week.

Strength training: Strength training assembles muscle mass, which can assist with helping digestion and burn calories even at rest. Center around practices that target significant muscle gatherings, for example, squats, rushes, push-ups, and weightlifting. Aim for at least two days of solidarity preparing each week.

High-intensity interval training (HIIT): HIIT includes short eruptions of extraordinary activity followed by brief times of rest. It very well may be more effective than consistent state cardio for consuming calories and expanding digestion. Instances of HIIT practices incorporate bouncing jacks, burpees, hikers, and runs.

Yoga or Pilates: These activities center around center strength, adaptability, and equilibrium, which can assist with further developing stance, forestall wounds, and diminish pressure. They can likewise assist with building muscle and burn calories.

Everyday movement: Normal actual work over the course of the day, for example, using the stairwell rather than the lift, stopping farther away from the entry, or doing family tasks, can likewise assist with burning calories and increment digestion.

Make sure to talk with a medical care supplier prior to beginning any activity

program, particularly in the event that
you have any ailments or wounds.

Section 2

Skipping meals can actually hinder weight loss efforts, especially for women. Here's how not skipping meals can help:

Helps Digestion: When you skip dinners, your digestion dials back to save energy, which can make it harder to get more fit. By eating consistently, your body realizes it will get the fuel it needs and keeps your digestion murmuring.

Prevents overeating: When you skip dinners, you're bound to indulge later in the day, which can prompt consuming a greater number of calories than your body needs. Eating routinely helps keep cravings under control and keeps you from overeating.

Assists Control With blooding Sugar Levels: Eating normal, adjusted dinners can assist with managing glucose levels, which can prevent desires and overeating. This is particularly significant for ladies, who might be more prone to insulin obstruction.

Gives Energy for Exercise: Skipping meals can leave you feeling drained and languid, making it harder to muster the nerve to work out. Eating standard meals gives your body the fuel it needs to ride out exercises and burn calories.

Generally speaking, eating normal, balanced meals can assist ladies with getting in shape by supporting digestion, preventing overeating, controlling sugar levels, and giving energy to work out.

Section 3

On the off chance that you are encountering overthinking connected with weight reduction, there are a couple of systems you can attempt to diminish your pressure and uneasiness:

Put forth practical objectives: At times, overthinking happens when you put forth unreasonable or overpowering objectives. Ensure your weight reduction objectives are feasible, and separate them into more modest, more sensible advances.

Center around the cycle, in addition to the result: Rather than continually agonizing over how much weight you have lost, center around the moves you are making to arrive. Partake in the excursion and commend the little triumphs en route.

Practice care: Care methods like profound breathing, contemplation, and yoga can assist with quieting your psyche and diminish pressure.

Track down help: Conversing with companions, family, or a specialist about your weight reduction excursion can assist with mitigating a portion of the strain and stress you might feel.

Get sufficient rest: Rest is significant for in general wellbeing, including weight reduction. Ensure you are getting sufficient rest to assist with diminishing pressure and work on your psychological wellness.

Keep in mind, overthinking can be a characteristic piece of the weight reduction process, however it means quite a bit to track down sound ways of overseeing it so you can keep on track and roused on your objectives.

Section 4

Eating heaps of fruits and vegetables can be useful for weight reduction in more than one way:

Low calorie thickness: Fruits and vegetables are by and large low in calories however high in fiber and water content, and that implies you can eat a ton of them without drinking an excessive number of calories. This can help you feel full and fulfilled while diminishing your general calorie consumption, which can prompt weight reduction.

Supplement thick: Products of the soil are likewise plentiful in nutrients, minerals, and other helpful supplements that are significant for generally speaking wellbeing. By integrating them into your eating regimen, you can guarantee that you are getting the supplements your body needs without consuming overabundance calories.

Decreased desires: Eating more products of the soil can likewise assist with lessening desires for unhealthy, high-fat food sources. This is on the grounds that they contain fiber and water, which can assist with keeping you feeling full and fulfilled for longer timeframes, lessening the probability of gorging or nibbling on undesirable food sources.

Better absorption: The fiber content in products of the soil can likewise assist with further developing assimilation and lessen swelling, which can cause you to feel lighter and more agreeable, particularly assuming you are inclined to stomach related issues.

In general, integrating more leafy foods into your eating regimen can be a useful procedure for weight reduction and by and large wellbeing. It's memorable's critical that weight reduction is an intricate interaction that includes many elements, and that a decent eating

routine and ordinary active work are
key parts of a sound way of life.

Section 5

Getting a decent night's rest can assume a critical part in weight reduction for ladies in more than one way:

Hormone regulation: Absence of rest can disturb the equilibrium of hormones that direct hunger and satiety, like ghrelin and leptin. Ghrelin invigorates hunger, while leptin signals fullness. At the point when you don't get sufficient rest, ghrelin levels increment, and leptin levels decline, which can prompt increased hunger and overeating.

Metabolic function: Rest likewise assumes a part in directing your digestion. Studies have demonstrated the way that deficient rest can prompt a decrease in metabolic rate, which can make it harder to get thinner.

Energy and inspiration: When you're sleepless, you might feel tired and need energy, which can make it harder to adhere to a sound eating regimen and work-out daily practice.

Stress decrease: Absence of rest can likewise increment feelings of anxiety, which can prompt gorging or going to unfortunate survival strategies.

To guarantee you're getting a decent night's rest, it's essential to lay out sound rest propensities, for example,

Laying out an ordinary rest schedule: Attempt to head to sleep and awaken simultaneously consistently.

Establishing a loosening up rest climate: Keep your room peaceful, cool, and dim, and limit screen time before bed.

Staying away from energizers: Stay away from caffeine, liquor, and nicotine before bed.

Overseeing pressure: Track down solid ways of overseeing pressure, like through   exercise   or   unwinding procedures.

By and large, getting a decent night's rest is a significant piece of a sound way of life and can assume a huge part in weight reduction for ladies.

Section 6

Reducing carbohydrates consumption can assist with weight reduction for ladies in more than one way:

Bringing down calorie consumption: Starches are a significant wellspring of calories in many individuals' eating regimens. By decreasing how much starches consumed, ladies can diminish their calorie admission, which can prompt weight reduction.

Bringing down insulin levels: Sugars can cause spikes in insulin levels, which can advance fat stockpiling. By lessening sugar utilization, insulin levels can be brought down, which can cause it more straightforward for the body to burn fat for energy.

Diminishing desires: Numerous ladies find that lessening their carbohydrates consumption can assist with decreasing desires for desserts and other high-carbohydrates food sources, which can make it simpler to adhere to a good dieting plan.

Expanding satiety: High-carbohydrates meals can frequently leave ladies feeling hungry not long after eating. By lessening starch utilization and expanding the admission of protein and solid fats, ladies can feel more full for longer timeframes, which can decrease generally calorie consumption.

It's essential to take note of that while lessening sugar utilization can be useful for weight reduction, keeping a effective and healthy diet is as yet significant. Ladies ought to talk with a medical services supplier or enlisted dietitian to decide the perfect proportion of starches for their singular requirements and objectives.

Section 7

Expanding protein consumption can assist with weight reduction for ladies in more ways than one:

Boosting metabolism: Protein has a higher thermic impact than carbohydrates or fat, and that implies that the body consumes a larger number of calories processing protein than it does processing other macronutrients. This can prompt a lift in digestion, which can assist with weight reduction.

Preserving lean muscle mass: When ladies get in shape, they can likewise lose muscle mass. Consuming more protein can assist with safeguarding muscle mass, which is significant for keeping a healthy metabolism and preventing weight recapture.

Section 8

Decreasing liquor intake can assist with weight reduction for ladies in more than one way:

Reducing calorie intake: Alcohols are in many cases high in calories, and lessening or killing them can essentially decrease your general calorie consumption. For instance, a 5-ounce glass of wine normally contains around 120 calories, and a 12-ounce brew can contain around 150-200 calories. Removing a couple of beverages each day can bring about a critical decrease in calorie consumption over the long run.

Further developed digestion: Drinking liquor can dial back your digestion, causing it harder to consume calories and get thinner. At the point when you decrease or dispense with liquor from your eating routine, your digestion might improve, permitting you to productively consume calories more.

Better food decisions: Drinking liquor can bring down your restraints and make you bound to pursue unfortunate food decisions. At the point when you diminish your liquor admission, you might find it more straightforward to settle on better food decisions, which can likewise assist with weight reduction.

Better rest: Liquor can disturb rest designs, which can prompt weakness and make it harder to adhere to smart dieting propensities. At the point when you diminish your liquor admission, you might find that you rest better and have more energy to adhere to your weight reduction objectives.

Generally, diminishing liquor admission can be a basic and successful method for supporting weight reduction endeavors for ladies. It's essential to take note of that liquor ought not be totally killed from your eating regimen, yet rather consumed with some restraint.

Section 9

Drinking sufficient water can help ladies in their weight reduction endeavors in more ways than one:

Builds sensations of completion: Drinking water previously and during meals can assist you with feeling more full, which might help you eat less and decrease calorie admission.

Supports digestion: Drinking water can expand your resting metabolic rate, the rate at which your body consumes calories very still. This can assist you with consuming more calories over the course of the day.

Assists with hydration: Dehydration can prompt exhaustion and decreased actual work, which can upset weight reduction endeavors. Drinking sufficient water guarantees that your body is appropriately hydrated, assisting you with feeling stimulated and bound to participate in active work.

Lessens fluid calorie consumption: Drinking water rather than fatty refreshments, for example, pop and squeeze can diminish by and large calorie admission and help weight reduction.

Helps digestion: Water helps keep the stomach related framework working appropriately, forestalling blockage and bulging that can cause you to feel awkward and beat active work down.

In general, drinking sufficient water can be a basic yet powerful device for ladies to help with their weight reduction endeavors. It can assist with lessening calorie consumption, increment digestion, help in processing, and further develop hydration levels, all of which can add to weight reduction achievement.